ONE FOOT FORWARD

Reflections
on healing

Milena
Cifali

First published in 2023 by Echo Books.

Echo Books is an imprint of Superscript Publishing Pty Ltd,
ABN 76 644 812 395

Registered Office: Registered Office: PO Box 669,
Woodend, Victoria, 3442.

www.echobooks.com.au

Creator: Cifali, Milena, Author

Title: One Foot Forward: reflections on healing

ISBN: 978-1-922603-19-7 (paperback)

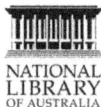

A catalogue record for this
book is available from the
NATIONAL
LIBRARY   National Library of Australia
OF AUSTRALIA

Book layout and design by Peter Gamble, Canberra
Set in Garamond Premier Pro Light Display, 12/15, and
MinervaModern.

All art in this book, including on the front cover, is original art
by Milena Cifali

echo))
BOOKS

CONTENTS

PREFACE

As I lay bruised and battered in my hospital bed in August 2022, I began writing out my pain, as I had previously done in my first book *Mallacoota Time*, written after the bushfires of the Australian summer of 2019–2020.

At that time my writing had been cathartic, and had not been designed to culminate in a book. I was simply writing to process my raw emotions.

Again, in hospital, some two years later, I began writing cathartically, to attempt to make sense of what had just occurred: in returning to my hometown of Mallacoota, Victoria after losing everything in the bushfires, to seek some closure, the return journey had instead culminated in my being rolled over by my own car and trapped, and ending up broken, in hospital. Some closure ...

When I finally returned home to Brisbane, the thoughts and emotions that had begun to emerge in my manuscript continued to evolve.

Like shards of broken ceramics, I began to piece them together, to create a series of small mosaics, with the central theme of healing.

I come not as a professional or expert on healing; I am merely the subject, the broken person that needs to be healed; I observe what has aided that healing and what has been counterproductive to that healing.

I do so in the sincere hope that others who may be suffering physical or emotional distress may find, within my words, some comfort and support.

If this occurs for even one person, then my trauma will have been worthwhile.

Milena Cifali

FOREWORD

When Milena reached out to ask me if I could preface her newest work I was humbled and felt the weight of the gift that she has given me.

These last few years in our collective history have been a journey from natural disaster, through the isolation of Covid, the fires, the floods, the separation of beliefs, the struggle to comprehend a shifting planet. It is through the eyes of artists that we can begin to comprehend this time, and move toward some type of reconciliation, and healing.

What *One Foot Forward* brings to this conversation is a symphony of bittersweet moments. It is a lament for all our sorrow. One cannot read this and not feel changed somehow. It is as though we too are trapped beneath a car; as though we too gaze through hospital windows at the beloved Brindabellas. We know these people within the hospital room because they are intrinsic reflections of ourselves and our own pain. We feel the strength of lost community, the sorrow of songs no longer sung, the fragility of life itself.

This story is a dichotomy of love and loss, hope and despair, putting into words those blurred moments as we walk through trauma and arrive at some foreign place where we drift without connection.

The lyrical soul of an artist who is poet, musician, painter and photographer is stripped bare through the experience of losing everything. A journey seeking closure and healing leads to yet more loss, more trauma and more pain.

In suffering we find life. In pain we find love. It is evident that from her personal struggles Milena has found the valuable gift of acceptance. That wondrous ability to be within the moment, noticing breath and stillness. With acceptance of our suffering comes true healing. Milena gives voice to our collective trauma that exists for some as a shrieking banshee and others a simmering tension. Within her words is the courage to heal, to face fear head on, to reach out and connect with others.

Beware then, as you read her words, to be confronted with raw pain and an uncanny knowing of our universal struggles. Hang in there though as the song of the beloved birds, the colours of this tormented land, the beauty of our simple connections and the overwhelming sense of love that has created this work changes you forever.

Kim Hollingshead
Registered Counsellor

Milena Cifali has been forced to learn a lot about healing in recent times. After her beautiful house in Mallacoota burned down in the Black Summer of 2019 (as recounted in her lyrical memoir *Mallacoota Time*), Milena moved to the comfort of her erstwhile community and people in Canberra with her partner

Jim for a couple of years. Milena explains in her earlier book that she was suffering from a sort of solastagia and searching for 'home', having become violently separated from her place in the world and her beloved animal friends. Canberra proved healing and Milena found comfort in old friends who made her and Jim feel supported, even as Jim had to undergo health challenges of his own. From here it was on to her lovely new beginning on the outskirts of Brisbane, and perhaps 'home'.

Tragically for a gifted and prolific composer and songwriter, only one song emerged for quite a while after the events of New Year's Day 2020, but in Brisbane Milena regained her voice and confidence, and a uniquely collaborative album followed. Milena premiered some of these new songs in Canberra and was determined to revisit Mallacoota to put to rest some ghosts of the past, and more than anything to take healing in the form of her new songs to the people she had lived with and loved in Mallacoota. This she was able to do (she rightly calls it a pilgrimage), and she was even able to come to terms in a way with the nothingness that met her where her old home in Mallacoota used to stand.

But fate had another twist in store for Milena when she returned to Canberra from Mallacoota, when her parked hire car rolled over her in somewhat bizarre circumstances, leaving her badly injured and unable to walk, though through sheer determination she is regaining that ability a little bit every day. *One Foot Forward* is the result of this mishap. Once again, Milena has transformed a personal tragedy into a message of hope and love, her mission to bring joy to the deeply traumatised and a renewed sense of meaning. In her inimitable lyrical style, she writes:

Sometimes you get what you least expect
You might not know it, but it might be for the best
Sometimes life throws you a test
Might not know it but it might be for the best.

This speaks to our many experiences in life of developing the patience and courage to see ourselves through the dark times that are part of the human condition.

One Foot Forward weaves back and forth between Milena's experiences of loss over the past few years, interspersed with acutely observed (and sometimes heartrending) accounts of moments in the often impersonal settings of the hospital. Even here, there are moments of grace, from a kindly nurse to connecting on a deeply human level with Freya, a young woman whose seemingly incurable and unbearably painful condition is matched by her determination to find purpose and joy. Milena finds time even here to sing or play people her songs, and some are moved to tears and tell her how healing it was for them.

There are sharply drawn vignettes reflecting on the grand themes of life: time and memory (childhood), the essentials of life (food, movement, breath) and the emotions that accompany them (laughter and crying). And of course, family and home, which we always circle back to when all is done. And the miracle of nature is never far from Milena's thoughts—you might say that in a sense this provides the scaffolding for everything Milena writes and sings about (water, sunlight, honey, flora and fauna).

In the span of a few short pages, Milena provokes us to look deeply at our lives and work on healing ourselves, our relationships with each other, and of course with the earth whose suffering and anguish reflects our own. In undertaking the sort of healing journey so wonderfully signposted by Milena in *One Foot Forward*, each of us might at last find our way Home, and thus find that in spite of all its challenges the journey was worthwhile after all.

Ranjan Chadhauri
Editor

I dedicate this book to my sons, Bryn and Louie, and my grandchildren, Willow, Violet and Tully.

I also write these words for all striving to heal from trauma; I hope somewhere within these pages you find the inspiration to put one foot forward. One step at a time...

Love
Heals all things
Believes all things
Hopes all things
Endures all things
1 Corinthians 13:7

A MISHAP

Flying home. Yes, home, that place where everything is just so. Moreton Bay unfolding from my aircraft window, a tapestry of turquoise, aqua, indigo, rippling gold: ethereal abstract geometry. I want to paint it. This is my new world.

One of vibrant green bamboo, clear blue skies, tropical flowers on steroids, of a world painted purple at jacaranda time, and splattered in red when summer poinsettias bloom. My mind casts back to the big drought of 2019. Yellow, black, smoky, grey. Drab.

Everything was drying, dying...

Snap back to reality. A butcher bird lands in the rich bamboo foliage and flies away to sparkling eucalypts against a chalk blue sky. The fires and loss of our home in Mallacoota in 2019 now diminished, painted out by brilliantly coloured brushstrokes: a new, lush environment. I dream in emerald and sapphire...

Emerald And Sapphire Dreams
When life has got you down
You might not see
the colours around
You might see life in black and white
And all your days turn to night
But give it time you'll see it's true
The colours will come back to you
The green and blue
Shining through
Heart in tune with blue and green
Never in my wildest dreams
Have I seen a blue as blue
A green as green
Today, today it's clear it's real
This is the way I want to feel
I'm settling down
looking around
feet on the ground
finally found
Attuned to all of nature's sounds ...
The green and blue
The blue and green
Never in my wildest dreams ...
Sky blue Leaf green
emerald and sapphire dreams
emerald and sapphire dreams...
I am fortunate to have survived.

My rental hybrid car rolled over me, as I got out to get my luggage, dragging me down the driveway and rolling onto my right foot. Trapped.

Lying in the driveway, in the Canberra drizzle, seconds after a spectacular sunset, wondering how the car has come to a stop. The only thing preventing it from rolling further: my foot. Dazed, trying to think how to remove myself from this terrifying, painful situation. Hoping the car does not gain momentum, continue rolling over me.

I left our home in Brisbane to fly to Canberra in late winter of 2022. Filled with hope, purpose and excitement. Two goals: my first foray back into music performance (after a creative drought brought on by Covid restrictions and dislocation after the fires), and a pressing need to return to Mallacoota to seek closure.

For a year and a half, I had felt an escalating sense of being in exile. A feeling of entrapment on The Island of Queensland. Restrictions had made it impossible to travel. I was disconnected from community, friendship. My time had now come to right this situation, so with the easing of restrictions, I took the plunge. I would return to Mallacoota.

Flying into Canberra, observing the muted golds and khaki greens of patchwork paddocks, I felt a sense of arrival in another land. This land, one I knew intimately, had been my childhood home, as well as cocooning me snugly in 2020, when we relocated here after the bushfires in Mallacoota. Canberra: here I could reconnect with friends forged over a lifetime, some who were in fact as much aunts and cousins as friends.

Here also were a network of musicians, most with whom I had performed in my past, and with whom there existed creative rapport. It was a place where I could navigate its parameters without the need of a map. As the aircraft touched down on the tarmac, I was, in a sense, home.

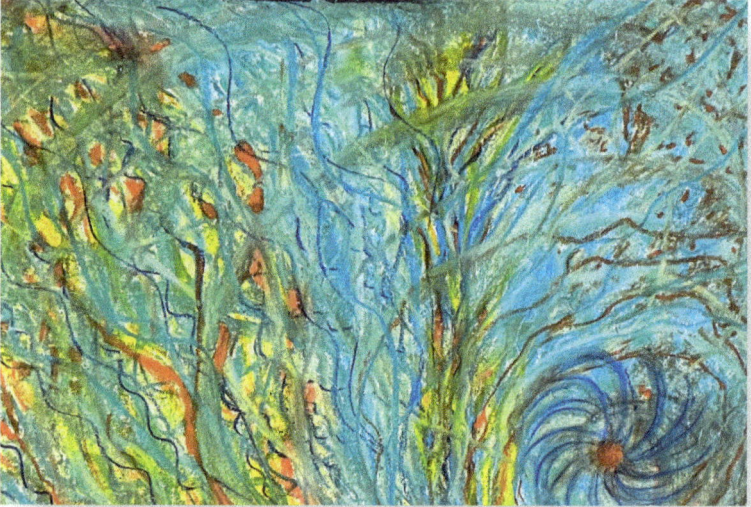

Emerald and sapphire dreams

CREATIVITY

For two years, since 2020, I had experienced a creative drought: unable to write music. The loss of my guitars, compositions, collection of sheet music acquired over almost a lifetime; CDs, my recordings, the loss of our performance life and musical community had been too much to bear. In that year I had written one song, 'Days Roll By'.

It was one little teardrop.

With our move to Brisbane in 2021, creativity begins to unfold; the lazy humidity and mild balmy breezes gradually relax the body, mind and spirit. I write songs about my new environment, laments over the loss of home and wildlife in Mallacoota, songs of hope, and love. A rekindling occurs -I feel a spark to connect musically with others.

I decide to record an album. The process is unlike any I have undergone before. Previously, I had performed in the studio with other musicians, and an album was usually completed within a few weeks. Now the experience is essentially solitary; it involves arriving at the recording studio to play guitar and sing. With the sound engineer at his desk, and myself alone, door closed, with only the microphone for company, I sing and play my songs, to be permanently duplicated. I emerge, to listen and evaluate the result with the sound engineer.

Within two days I complete my task. The digital files are then sent to the contributing musicians. The file then returns, for me to listen to. Each time, it feels like unwrapping a gift; this is always filled with excitement. The entire process takes over six months.

In creating my new album, *This Is Now*, I want to link my past life in Canberra and the South Coast with my present in Brisbane. So, I choose musicians from Canberra, (some whom I have known since childhood), and musicians from Brisbane, (whom I have never met), to collaborate with. I make an instant friend in Brisbane at my book launch for *Mallacoota Time* at the Logan Art Gallery. The connection is immediate and that is that. She is a photographer and graciously undertakes a photo shoot on my leafy balcony one afternoon. This becomes the front cover of my album. The back cover photography is shot by a renowned Canberra photographer; the connection between past and present on *This Is Now* complete.

I *am on stage. Finally. Under lights. A guitar in hand. Fingers poised over frets.*

The audience before me ...

Here is my sense of purpose; everything is right with the world. Just so. This is where I belong. I am like an athlete at the start line before the gun fires. Filled with anticipation and adrenalin. The audience in the bohemian lounge room setting, Smiths, is filled with familiar faces: some I have known for forty years, others only four. I know they are here out of love and support, as are the musicians joining me onstage. I feel blessed.

I speak from the heart to this beautiful audience, of my love for music, my grief, my healing journey. And the music begins. Two hours, or a lifetime. Baring my soul intimately. A friend whose daughter went missing one day over twenty years ago and never returned, comes to tell me how my songs have helped her tonight. I hug and talk to people, many people, from various parts of my life. This is my pilgrimage from desert to oasis. A feast of friendship, of human connection.

I am overwhelmed. Grateful. Tired. I sleep soundly. My alarm is set to drive the winding road from Canberra to Mallacoota in the morning.

MALLACOOTA: THE RETURN

Six in the morning. I am awake and ready to travel to the South Coast. This road, to Bungendore, where my father worked the Lake George area as a geologist during my childhood, so familiar, and then the approach to Braidwood, where I have stopped innumerable times over the years for coffee, antique fossicking and birthday celebrations. Then the road out, Poplar Road, also the title of one of my songs on my previous album. This stretch of road always represented a halfway point in my trip to the beach as a child. Poplar road was the place where I would roll my window down and gulp in the air (sensing I could smell the ocean), where my child's heart did a somersault at the thought of crashing waves, golden sand and fish and chips.

Then, the winding U-turns past Pooh Corner, snaking down to Batemans Bay. Now, I see through burnt-out forest, still blackened after two years, a hint of ocean on the horizon below. How I have achingly missed this coast, my second home, since arriving in Brisbane! I cross the new bridge to Batemans Bay, stop to absorb the familiar view, that calm blue bay punctuated by small rocky islands, then stopping again at Denham's Beach, where my partner Jim and I have spent so many nights in our

Oka, waking to a pale pink day on our regular trips along the coast from Mallacoota to perform music.

I drive onwards to Moruya, the town where I had my first family holiday in Australia when I was almost too little to remember. I make an obligatory stop, as we always have done, at the Monarch Hotel, not for a drink, but to visit our beautiful friend Donald, the sulphur crested cockatoo. I am bursting with excitement at the prospect. I have so missed him. I arrive, but do not spot him. My heart sinks. With a start I realise he might have passed away. I walk toward the car, and then I see him:

Donald. I am overjoyed! The poor bird lives alone, and is often reserved, daydreaming, remembering better times perhaps, but I usually manage to liven him up and have a conversation. When I leave, he always screams, 'bye bye! bye bye!'. Poor Donald. I feel sad as I drive away. I might not have the opportunity to visit Donald for another year or two. He might not even be here next time ... .

There is no time to stop in Narooma, with its jewelled turquoise waters, a place we have played music frequently, camping near the rock wall, falling asleep to the crashing waves so many times. Narooma is a familiar old friend. Before the approach to Tathra, I meander on through the cathedral-like spotted gum forest, a magnificent, iconic part of the South Coast landscape. The tall trees welcome me back. How many times we have travelled this enchanting stretch of road.

I turn off the Highway towards Bermagui, a place that has been a constant backdrop to my life: a place that I have holidayed as a young woman with my mother, for quality mother daughter time; the place where I met the love of my life, Jim; a place where we have performed music, where the community has become our community. I have arranged to meet a few friends at the Bermagui Hotel.

The interlude is short, sweet and strong, a shot of espresso. A refuelling of friendship. I stay overnight with friends to rest and am up early again for the return to Mallacoota. I need closure.

How Do I Say Goodbye?

New Year's Eve our home burnt down
Leaving ash upon the ground
Blackened trees devoid of life
Where once the magpies sang.
Remembering the golden light
And lorikeets in coloured flight
Three billion creatures died that day
The memory won't fade away
How do I say goodbye
To sunny Mallacoota skies
Where eagles soared up high
makes me want to cry
Sunset clouds gelato hues
Endless ocean vivid blues
Morning walks on golden sand
Tiny shells in palm of hand
How do I say goodbye
To magic Mallacoota nights
Where moon shine silver on the sea
Takes away the heart of me
I'll start again
I'll move on
But forever I will sing this song

My Mallacoota melody
Makes me want to cry.
New Year's Eve our home burnt down
leaving ash upon the ground
Blackened trees devoid of life
Where once magpies sang
How do I say goodbye
to sunny Mallacoota skies
Where eagles soared up high
Makes me want to cry
How do I say goodbye
Makes me want to cry
How do I say goodbye.

Monday 22 August 2022

The road home. Home to Mallacoota. But there is no home. Our cottage and everything in it was destroyed by the New Year's Eve bushfires of 2019. I want to try and lessen the traumatic memories I have been scarred with, upon seeing our beautiful home reduced to rubble, on national television on New Year's morning. And then, a few weeks later, a thickening of scarring, brought about by the horrific experience of a brief return visit to Mallacoota on 8 February 2020, where I stood before the ash, attempting to make sense of what I witnessed: our melted twisted bird cage that once harboured our vibrant feathered friends: blackened trees where once magpies sang; the town smelling of rain drenched ash, an eerie grey ghost town. Silent. On that day I had fled, engulfed by anxiety.

I am here again to seek closure. I have butterflies in my stomach as I drive toward the town, trying to prepare mentally for what I might encounter. I have attempted to visualise what 11 Betka Road might look like now. I hope I am prepared. I pull into the main street, exit the car and stand for a few moments. Am I really here? It is surreal. I see familiar faces passing by. There are smiles, hugs, waves. I am back, with my community, that have endured too much...

Tuesday 23 August 2022—reflections upon leaving Mallacoota...

Oh Mallacoota, I fell in love with you all over again: your beauty, gentleness, wilderness, softness, even the blackened tea tree against the fluffy white clouds. Crying at the beauty the moment I arrived in Mallacoota, the view flooring me as my eyes met the vast expanse of silver blue, the Mallacoota inlet leading out to sea. The gentle waves caressing the golden expanse of limitless sand. I had walked that sand so many times, to the edge of the earth; or so it seemed...

Stepping out of my car upon arriving in Mallacoota, I was greeted by a seagull, who stared at me, stepping forward to welcome me, a true Mallacoota local. The people, and smiles. Hugs: some fleeting, tentative, caused by two years of Covid isolation; some long, lingering and warm, some as though the person hugging me was drowning—clinging for life.

I had lunch with the music teacher from the high school and with Padma the violinist, and another friend who plays percussion and bass. I was within my community once again, and people understood what our loss meant, as they had experienced it also. It felt grounding. I had felt anonymous in Brisbane for quite some time now and to be recognized and understood felt like a small miracle.

I drove to Betka Beach, walked through the burnt tea tree scrub, stark black against the white clouds, landing at the lookout which overlooks the wild coastline. I stilled my heart and soaked in the beauty I could have drowned in its splendour. I went to Captain Stephenson's lookout, always my favourite spot in Mallacoota, marvelling once more at the sight in front of me, which had become hazy in my mind's eye over time; now reappearing with razor sharp clarity, knocking me off my feet. A watercolour poem ...

I went to the community hall, known as The Muddy and Padma, beautiful hearted soul, had organised a community music night. I have played here many times with Jim. I once again smiled at the people of Mallacoota, and shared my soul through a few songs, against the backdrop of a Mallacoota bird painting while Padma created Magic with his violin strings, his bow creating a tapestry rich and sweet, embroidering my music with love.

I stayed with my neighbours, Robyn and Bill, whose house had also burnt down. They had since rebuilt. I tried to fathom how the empty block next door, which once used to be our home, was now a vacant, muddy space, with only a caravan on it, and not one tree. I could not make sense of it, so I gave up trying. Still, I missed the idea of being able to simply walk to my front door, go inside, make a cup of tea and sit on the balcony, on our old blue couch, to once again listen to the waves...

Robyn and Bill nurtured me, made me dinner, gave me a comfortable bed. In the morning I woke at 6am to drizzle. I went to Bastion Point to survey the wild grey ocean. Once again, the stunning landscape, today a sombre and moody oil painting, took my breath away: the soft muted misty hues, rolling waves, and even the blackened tea tree scrub framing it: my heart skipped a beat.

At 6.30am I pulled into Gaz's driveway to see him for a cup of coffee by his fire. He was one of those, who, like me, had lost his home. He played me the cello, his bow skimming light as a feather over the strings. He had only been learning for six months but I could sense the beauty, the transparency, the lightness of touch. He is a musician. He is also an artist. Gaz showed me his newly built art studio and the blank cobalt blue canvases, silently and expectantly waiting to become expressions of art from his soul. He told me that in loss there are often almost always blessings to be found: *but you have to look for them*.

In making the pilgrimage back to Mallacoota, I feel that this was exactly what I was doing. Albeit for such a short time, I was able to receive its gifts and hopefully give some back through my music, a smile, a hug. I am blessed to have returned, for in doing so I was able to reduce those traumatic memories of the day I fled the bleak blackness on 8 February 2020, replacing them with beauty, music, community, and the sharing of stories: ultimately another step towards healing.

Farewell, my Mallacoota. I shall return. I don't know how, or when, but return I will, to appreciate your gifts, perhaps share some of mine. Thank you. I am blessed; every step I take leads me towards healing, completion. For healing is a journey to be savoured, not a destination. Yes, I would have liked to stay, bask in

your glory for another day, week, year... But you will still be here;
I will return.

I have had time to think about the Mallacoota community;
my impression is that they are suffering collective trauma.
The trauma of standing under blood red skies, the fear of the
approaching flames, the blackened loss; the almost immediate
cessation of community connection due to Covid lockdowns;
the reality of an ashen town that could not be quickly rebuilt due
to a delay in tradespeople accessing the town; its geographical
remoteness. I have a clear sense that the beautiful strong
community that had existed previously is somehow frozen,
fractured and split. This makes me sad. The forest is regenerating
but the community may take longer to do so...

I want to return, listen and share stories, play music, connect.
I want to bring joy.

What Can I Bring

What can I bring to this life?
A song or four, an open door, an open heart
What can I bring to this day?
A song to play, three words to say,
three words to say...
Look above at the blue sky
stop and smell the yellow flowers
feel the rain on your skin
open your eyes and drink it all in...
I want to thank you for bringing this day,
I don't know who to thank but thank you anyway
What can I bring to your day

A friendly hug, a cosy rug,
to wrap us in, to wrap us in...
Look above at the blue sky
stop and smell the yellow flowers
feel the rain on your skin
open your eyes and drink it all in...

HOSPITAL

So, Mallacoota revisited, my plan is to drive back to Canberra for a restful night, then fly home to Brisbane and reflect on my experiences. But no. Plans have a way of being rewritten. Instead, I am trapped under my rental car. It is horrific and traumatic. I realise, after a few minutes, that my mobile phone is reachable. I call my friend whose driveway I am in. My friend and her partner materialise, to witness me splayed across the ground under the car. 'Can you please try and lift the car off my foot?' I say slowly, taking care to ensure I do not panic. Their attempts are in vain.

They gather around the car and attempt to lift it. No success. Excruciating pain. 'Can you please go to the back of the car and try to push it forward?' I am surprised by the evenness in my voice. In reality I am scared I might die. The car remains stationary. My foot, crushing under the tyre. Everything hurts.

I have had enough.

'Can you please try driving the car forward a metre or two?' Finally, the car rolls off my foot. I am freed. I attempt to rise and walk. My hip feels as though it has turned inside out. My ribs are crushing with pain. I remember that I am on blood thinners and decide to be driven to the hospital. After being wheeled into emergency, I am assessed at triage. I am then parked to wait. Wait ...during this time, the world fades in and out, becomes unreal; I have a strange auditory experience as though I am in a cave; I feel anxious. I am going to pass out. I call for help. A nurse arrives to take my blood pressure. It is very low. I am transferred to a bed, wheeled off for X-rays and CT scans. The cold glass hurts as I try to position myself for the scans. *Everything hurts. Everything.*

The doctor arrives hours later—it could be morning but here there is no morning, no sense of time. My right hip is broken. I am wheeled sometime in the middle of the following night to another ward. Fifth floor, bed 12C. Another set of crisp white sheets. There is a young man singing himself to sleep, self-soothing, in great pain.

'Scotty, come on Scotty' he whimpers softly. 'You can do it Scotty, oh my god Scotty'. Scotty continues this self-pleading throughout the night. I get no sleep whatsoever, save a few fitful minutes snatched here and there.

MOUNTAINS

On my new album is a song titled 'Brindabella Dreaming'. These mountains, which frame Canberra, have been a constant backdrop to my life.

Brindabella Dreaming

My Brindabella ranges of opalescent hues
Of stunning inky violet and watercolour blues
Of fire painted sunsets that turn the fields to gold
Of tendril misted valleys on mornings bright and cold
I love your constant presence, your spiritual essence
My Brindabellas whisper ancient Ngunnawal meaning
The ancestors aligning with my Brindabella dreaming
My Brindabella dreaming
My Brindabella dreaming the Milky Way above
My Brindabella dreaming the mountains that I love
My Brindabella Dreaming imprinted in my soul
My Brindabella Dreaming when I look at you, I'm home...

I wake in my hospital bed to see the Brindabellas in the morning sunlight. I am grateful for the view.

I hurt all over; their presence is comforting. Over the coming nights I am treated to an array of fire painted sunsets over the Brindabellas. They help to ease my pain.

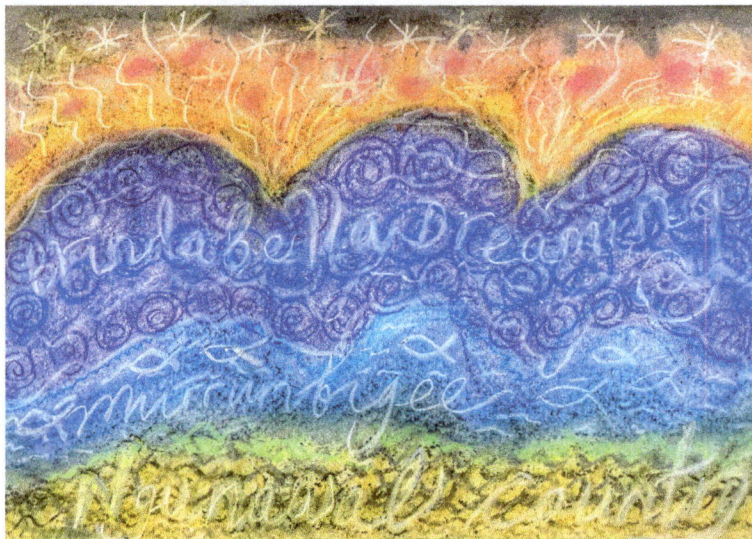

Brindabelle dreaming

MUSIC

There is a woman in the bed directly next to mine who cries in agony. She is experiencing tremors, trouble walking and heart problems. She and Scotty are very sick. One day we begin conversing. They learn that I am a musician and songwriter and ask how they can hear my music. I play 'Game's Not Over' through my phone, holding it up so they can hear it. The lady in the bed next to me says 'Thank you, I love your song. It has given me the strength to continue.' I feel a lump in my throat. She begins to cry. I begin to cry. Scotty begins to cry. We cry together. I do not know why I am here, in this hospital, with a broken hip, but perhaps, just perhaps, I am here for this moment.

Games Not Over
Sometimes you feel you're walking
backwards through life,
the very thing you think you're heading for
gets further away
sometimes you feel
the path you're on
is heading to a place you have to be,
but suddenly there's a fork
and you end up in a place you've never been

One door closes, another one opens,
Key's in your pocket, the games not over,
One door closes, another one opens,
Key's in your pocket the games not over,
One door closes another one opens....
Sometimes you feel like all is lost,
You've lost your way
And you don't know how to find a way to get back home,
You're feeling lost, and all alone.
Sometimes you get what you least expect
You might not know it, but it might be for the best
Sometimes life throws you a test
Might not know it but it might be for the best.
Sometimes you feel you're walking backwards through life
The very thing you think you're heading for gets further away
Sometimes you feel like all is lost you've lost your way
And you don't know how to find a way to get back home
You're feeling lost and all alone
One door closes another one opens
Key's in your pocket the game's not over
One door closes another one opens
Key's in your pocket the game's not over
One door closes another one opens ...

Music swirls, caresses, heals: Fills sick cells and renews them. Music can guide patients into meditation, relax sick children, ease the passage of a dying person, alter one's mood from stress to peace. It can provide hope where none exists; it can alleviate trauma, as my songs did for my friend whose daughter went missing... as it did today for two sick people in hospital.

Music gives wings to those who cannot fly.

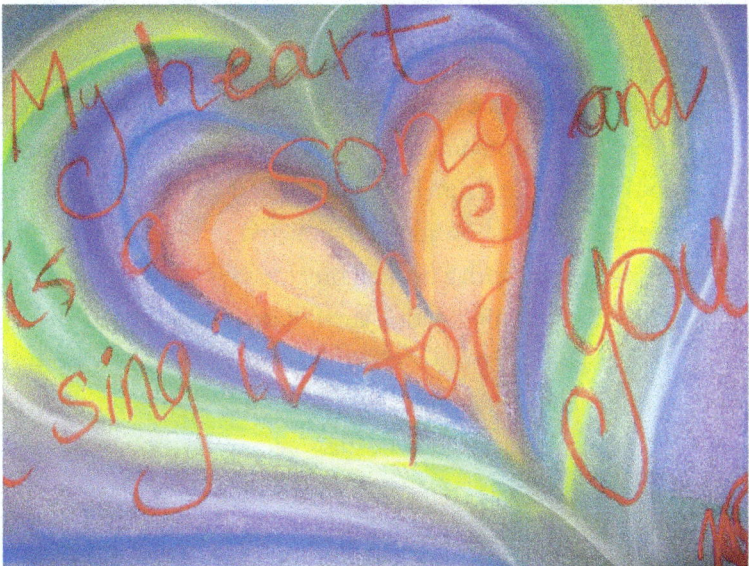

Music

A HARP

Today I receive a visit from the Pastoral Care team at the hospital. The man sits and talks with me for a while. I tell him about Jim's stroke three weeks before the bushfires, about losing our home, birds, instruments. About our move to Canberra. Then to Brisbane. I tell him how this trip was to be about healing but instead I am in a hospital bed, covered in black bruises and bleeding abrasions, with a broken hip. He says he has something that may help, returning with a small harp. I lay it gently on my chest, begin to play, to pluck the strings, the sound vibrating through my cells. I gradually relax, and the people in the ward seem to quieten also. A small healing occurs.

———

Abruptly, or so it seems, I am moved from my ward with the Brindabella view, and wheeled to another ward: the same, but different. Here, in bed 12D, my view is of the bathroom. A Sudanese woman, a study in contrast against the stark white sheets, is groaning and writhing, her head rolling this way and that. The woman opposite me is colouring in children's colouring books and speaking in a voice too loud for this time of the night. The bed which I now occupy vibrates to prevent pressure sores.

Rather than providing comfort, it makes me anxious, as though I have pins and needles all over...

After the sudden change of leaving Mallacoota due to the fires, the move to Canberra for a year, then the move to Brisbane, any move for me feels difficult, fraught with tension. This one is no better. I lay there, tensely, listening to the groaning woman, wishing I was back upstairs with my sunsets. I sleep for half an hour, and wake in the morning tearful, fragile and anxious.

I call a social worker, desperate to be moved to a quieter ward with a window. As the day progresses, I talk to my roommates and, as I begin to get to know them, I start to relax a little. I ask the nurses to make sure my view of the bathroom involves keeping the bathroom door closed as much as possible.

In the light of day, I can see sky, clouds and a few trees from the window across the room; these bring me comfort.

FREYA

Freya, you break my heart. I have come to be close to you over these fifteen days and nights, lying in the hospital bed next to yours, with only a curtain separating us, sometimes open, sometimes closed.

You are seventeen, fair skinned, with a Norwegian reddish blonde mane of hair. You love pizza, art and architecture. Your dream is to move to Japan to live, and you are already taking steps by learning the language. You are a cat lover and would like to own a bulldog. Your face lights up when your boyfriend comes to visit. You love to draw. Your life lays ahead of you, and you are filled with dreams and aspirations.

You cannot walk. You drag yourself, pushing a walker with jerking, spasmodic movements, your wasted leg muscles skinny white sticks. You cannot swallow and are on a liquid diet. You have lost five kilos since being here. You have been in and out of hospital for almost two years. You have had eight bleeding noses since I have been here. Your hair is falling out. You have undergone test upon test, and still, nobody knows what is wrong with you. You cry for hours in pain, but no one comes to help.

Nurses and doctors come and go, but rarely do they speak to you with empathy or kindness, rather asking perfunctorily where the pain is, and to tell them your name and date of birth. Still, you have a beautiful smile.

A psychiatrist comes in and tells you that your symptoms are all in your mind. She wants to put you on anti-psychotic medication, but you tell her you do not need it or want it. We have long conversations at night, and I tell you to remember that autonomy over your body is yours. A neurologist comes in and you plead for a test you have read about, for a disease that matches all your symptoms. The neurologist tells you it is unavailable and is a waste of taxpayer's money. You tell me, crying, that if they do not diagnose your problem soon, and just send you home on opiates, in a wheelchair, you will end up palliative, with no hope. 'They will send me home to die!' My heart breaks again. You are seventeen! Your whole life lays before you, Freya!

———

Today Freya is groaning and jerking spasmodically on the bed. She is on oxygen. She is crying out for help, to relieve the relentless pain gnawing at her stomach, ribs and back. A nurse comes, asks where the pain is, and comes back with pain killers. Still, she cries out. In the afternoon, Freya's nose starts to bleed. She is lying down, unable to swallow properly. The curtain is open. I press the buzzer for the nurse. The nurse arrives, props her up a little, dabs at the blood and leaves. Now it is flowing, spurting. Freya is gurgling.

'I'm choking on my blood! Help me!' No one is coming. She begins to spasm, having a seizure right in front of me. The nurse returns and calls a code red alert for medical staff. Suddenly, there are five, six doctors and five nurses in the room, all looking anxious, ready to act. A bright red resuscitation trolley is wheeled in.

'Freya! Freya! Can you open your eyes? Freya! Can you hear me?' Freya is nonresponsive. Freya has gone to another place. I am distressed, thinking she may die now, in the bed next to me. Her mother and father arrive, pacing, traumatised. After ten minutes the doctors and nurses leave. I get up to talk to Freya, who appears to be sleeping very deeply.

'It's ok Freya, you'll be ok. I'm here Freya.' She nods, almost imperceptibly. But it is a response. She has heard me. Freya's mother is pacing anxiously. 'She can still hear you' I say. 'Maybe talk to her.' Her mother goes to Freya's bedside 'I am here baby; mama is here Freya'. The visitors have left, and alone in the semi-dark of the ward, amongst the beeping machines, I am left to unravel my distress at what I have witnessed. I slow my breath, try to get some sleep.

TIME

There is an unwritten rule: when a friend or even an acquaintance ends up in hospital, the thing to do is to visit. Because of covid restrictions, I am allowed only two visitors per day for fifteen minutes each. Visitors come bearing gifts. Kalamata olives, a jar of vegemite, camomile hair mist and hairbrush, earplugs, citrus tarts, flowers, berries and chocolate. I sit up and try to make conversation. After fifteen minutes I am exhausted. But I know they come with support and love, as they did to my album launch a few days earlier. They have given the greatest gift one can give another: time. Kindness and care heals. To give time is to give love. I give thanks.

LISTENING

A young man comes to see me from Pastoral care. He is doing a Master's in Counselling and listens attentively to my story. He was brought up by a devout Anglican mother, but now has steered toward Buddhism. We discuss spirituality, what binds all faiths together: we concur that at their essence is the principle of loving thy neighbour, doing unto others as you would have done unto yourself, acting with kindness, being of service. It is Saturday. This young man could be playing golf in the sunshine. Instead, he is sitting by the beds of sick people, talking with them. Listening. Helping them heal.

NOT LISTENING

My foot is blue, grazed and swollen. I cannot move it. My ribs hurt. Breathing, moving, yawning and turning hurt. My abrasions and bruises hurt. My heart hurts. I do not understand why my healing trip has ended this way. I am an emotional roller coaster. My moods change every hour. I try to make everyone on the ward happy, I smile, joke, try and remain positive. On my way to the bathroom, being pushed in the wheelchair, I feel fragile and begin to cry. It is this way each day. The social worker comes to visit again. She does not say much but explains to me about complex trauma: layer upon layer of trauma, that if not kept in check can lead to various problems such as alcohol dependence. This makes me feel anxious. She leaves. I feel worse and more alone.

FAITH

Today, a third visit from Pastoral Care. This time a small, softly spoken Vietnamese woman. Her name is Kim. She sits and I want to speak but instead I begin to cry. Tears flow. Kim does not say much, just allows me to be in this space. She is from a mixed faith background, Catholic and Buddhist. We discuss the essence of faith, settling on love. 'To spread the love' she says. Yes.

A poem from my hospital bed
Sprinkle the love
Spread the love
Sow the love
Be the love
Be Love

She asks if she may pray for me. The prayer is heartfelt. I close my eyes and enter the spirit. I feel my first sense of peace since being trapped under that car. I play her one of my songs, the one called Game's Not Over; she listens intently, eyes closed. She tells me that she never thought she would be here, in a hospital, by people's bedsides, speaking with and helping them, as she is a shy and reserved person. She does it well; gently, softly, allowing much space for healing. Some nurses or doctors could learn much from her approach. Kim returns with a small gift for me: a wooden cross, all smooth and curved, like an ocean pebble. It fits in my hand perfectly and brings me comfort.

> *If I speak in the tongues of men and of angels but do not have love, I have become sounding brass or a clanging cymbal*

1 Corinthians 13:1

TOUCH AND EMPATHY

There is one nurse I will never forget. Her name is Rosemary. What sets Rosemary apart is her empathy. When she asks me in the early morning, 'How are you feeling?' She means it, allowing space for my answer. In the still of the night, she gives my hand a little squeeze. That little squeeze is love. That little squeeze is healing.

That little squeeze is everything.

NUTRITION

In the ward is a lady with the reddest, most swollen hand and arm I have ever seen. She is on intravenous antibiotics. She calls the nurse every hour: ' can I have a coffee? Eight sugars.'

I question if I have heard correctly. Eight sugars. She drinks five coffees in the space of the day. Forty sugars. Sometimes she takes her coffee downstairs to enjoy with a cigarette. I wonder how forty sugars laced with nicotine will help her swollen infected arm. I wish I could say something to help her, but I say nothing ...

Hospital food is alright. It does the job of keeping one fed. There is the obligatory scoop of reconstituted mashed potato and the regulation serve of frozen vegetables, just over-cooked. Meat or chicken in some unidentifiable sauce. Jelly, custard, ice cream and endless cups of tea. My friend brings three punnets of berries. Blueberries, blackberries, and raspberries. I open the raspberries to have one or two: the vibrant, juicy tang bursts in my mouth refreshing and awakening my senses. Before I realise it, the punnet is empty. I feel vitality permeating my cells, replenishing, healing.

SLEEP

I am awoken abruptly at 2am.

'Milena! Milena! It's time for your Panadol Milena!'

I wake with a start, a rush of anxiety. I was asleep! I was not in pain. I was awoken from deep slumber, one of the most necessary and healing forces known in nature; woken to take a man-made chemical. Please! Allow me two hours of sleep rather than two Panadol. Please!

MOVEMENT

Our bodies are designed to move. Our bodies dance, bend, flow. Physical activity has a profound impact on healing, both mental and physical. Even in hospital, bed bound, I make sure I am wiggling my toes, stretching my arms, doing ankle rolls. Longevity is linked to being active.

In cultures around the world where populations age well into long life, there appears to be a correlation between remaining active and productive, and longevity; harvesting crops, looking after grandchildren; studies show dementia can be kept at bay by physical activity. Breathe, stretch to the stars, bend like a tree, dance like a child, play. If these activities cause too much pain, undertake them in a heated pool, or in the ocean. I will be back in the pool, in my element, swimming, walking, gliding, breathing, bending, mending, as soon as I possibly can.

LAUGHING

In the hospital ward exists much suffering: the lady across from me has lost her sister today, her last remaining sibling out of nine. She is unable to attend the funeral as she is too ill. Last year she lost her daughter, and grandson. Freya is writhing in pain, unable to eat or sleep. Robyn sits, sadly and silently colouring to fill her bleak days. I also suffer, unable to turn, cough or move because of the excruciating pain in my ribs. I feel the pain of those around me. This hurts me also.

I try to help the others in the ward laugh, and they do. I make jokes, and the nurses laugh also. I laugh at myself, mostly. 'I will start dancing in a moment if you are not careful!' I say, as they watch me take my first four, tentative, shaky steps on crutches. 'Let's order lobster mornay tonight' I say to my ward mates, making them smile.

Laughter lessens pain, strengthens relationships, breaks the ice, promotes circulation, releases endorphins and boosts the immune system. The people of India have known this for centuries; they gather in parks across the land to practice laughter yoga. There now exist around five thousand intentional laughter clubs worldwide, across fifty-three countries. Laughter is one of the tools we may draw upon in our healing.

Laughter is medicine.

CRYING

A beautiful piece of music, or a nostalgic recollection can make one cry, as can grief, bringing out heart wrenching sobs. Homesickness may produce a single, silent tear, or memories of a love lost may make the eyes well. Crying is the body's natural response to deeply felt emotion. As adults we feel the need to apologise if we start to cry in front of someone else. Letting our boundaries and defences down is somehow unacceptable.

At the hospital, a few moments after making those around me laugh, I am transferring to a wheelchair to be pushed to the bathroom. Suddenly, my ribs catch with agonising sharpness. I feel helpless, a burden. I feel that my mobility may be impaired for a long time to come. I feel the poignancy of having returned to Mallacoota where we lost everything. The sadness at having left yet again. The joy and sweetness of finally playing music again; the cruelty of having that ripped away from me suddenly by this accident. I cry. I cry and cry. A floodgate has opened. Nurses and my ward mates are watching me: yet I have nothing to apologise for. Crying is a healthy and natural mechanism. Crying sets us free.

BIRD SONG

The auditory experience of the hospital is one of beeping machines, trolleys, and the hum of air-conditioning. One can become accustomed to these noises, and their ability to intrude on sleep or relaxation lessens as time goes by. There is no fresh air. The air is recycled and air-conditioned and most likely overheated. There is no natural light. The lights are on day and night; the overhead lights are overly bright.

Returning home, yes, home, I step into my bedroom and lay on my bed with pale blue sheets and ocean blue pillowcases. Not a stark white sheet in sight. My window is open. There is a gentle breeze wafting over me, smelling of sunlight and cut grass. My view is bamboo, vibrant, green, alive. Birds flitter amongst its foliage as do butterflies. When I sleep, the first night back in my own bed, the room is dark. I sleep like a baby; awake to a sunrise and the first thing I hear is birdsong. After hearing no birds, only the beeps of machines for sixteen days, it comes as a surprise to my ears: I am filled with a sense of gratitude to be back in the arms of the music of nature. Imagine a world without the song of birds ... .

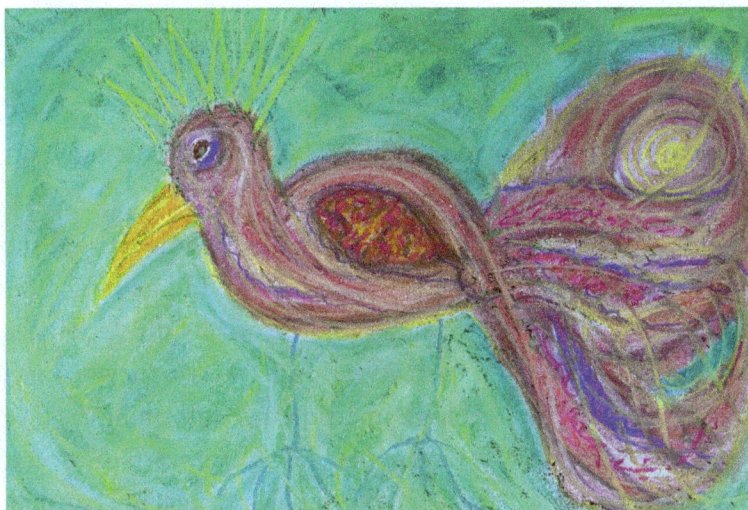

Birdy magic

HONEY

Bees are magical and mystical creatures. Their importance and sacredness are well documented through the aeons of history in ancient Babylonian, Hittite, Egyptian, Greek, Chinese and other civilisations. The folklore about bees form a substantial part of these cultures.

Honey and beeswax have been important products since the Mesolithic period. Bees are our pollinators and without bees quite simply, we would struggle and eventually die. Upon the honeybees' return to their hive with pollen for honey-making, bees perform an incredible geometric dance, informing the hive of the location of flowers and pollen. The bee converts the nectar into honey by secreting enzymes from their stomach. They then flap their little wings vigorously at very high speed to reduce moisture. It requires around four million flowers to make one kilogram of honey, and to do so the bee needs to fly distances of up to approximately 1600 kilometres. Bees are intelligent, look out for each other, dance and bees make a magical substance called honey.

There is evidence that honey was used as a medicinal

treatment for many ailments as far back as ancient Mesopotamia. Ancient Greeks named honey 'the food of the gods' and indeed it is. This liquid gold has many healing properties: It is anti-inflammatory, antibacterial, and soothing. It promotes healing of wounds when placed on the skin topically, and healing of the body when taken internally. Honey has antioxidant properties similar to many fruits and vegetables and is one of the only food sources known to mankind to never spoil, having an everlasting shelf-life.

Manuka honey in particular is prized for its exceptional healing properties. I asked my friend to bring me a pot of Manuka honey, and it is part of my daily ritual. I take a teaspoon in the morning and a teaspoon at night. My swollen blue foot that I have been unable to move begins to reduce in size after only two days of taking the honey. I am able to start wiggling my toes and start gently rotating my ankle. The honey begins to work its magic on my enormous, blackened bruises, and after two days they begin changing colour, becoming lighter.

The bees' well-being, and their continuation on this planet, is of utmost importance. We must honour and protect our bees. We are their caretakers. I give thanks to the bees.

PUSHKI

On 9 September 2021 exactly a year ago to the day I wrote these words, I decided to adopt a cat. I have always had cats and am a cat lover.

Whilst being the carers of birds is wonderful, having a cat around the home was something I really missed.

Today I am back in Brisbane, from the hospital, and my right rib is bruised and very painful. My cat Pushki must sense this: she comes and lies gently across my rib with her paws over my chest, her tummy over my sore rib, and purrs into the rib. The warmth and the vibration seem to relieve the pain and promote healing. She also lies against my broken hip; the warmth is healing.

When I feel stressed, tired or sick there is nothing more comforting than a purring cat on my lap. I slowly stroke her champagne silk fur. She gazes into my eyes with her deep blue ones. I feel content.

BREATH

The practice of meditation, which simply means going inwards, is one that has been used by many cultures since the beginning of time for reflection and healing. At its essence is an awareness of the breath.

At a pain management workshop a few years ago, I learnt that breathing in, then out for twice as long can promote well-being and lessen anxiety. It is a simple technique that I often rely on when feeling stressed or nervous. It can be done simply at any time of day for a minute or two. It can also help ease pain.

Whilst in the hospital one afternoon, talking to Freya, she was in agony. I went to her bedside, and I began to stroke her hand which was clenched like a dying bird's claw. I began to show her how to slow her breathing: slowly through the nose for a count of three and breathing out slowly through the nose for a count of six. She found it challenging because she was on oxygen, but it appeared to relax her. I then guided her through a meditation referred to as Yoga Nidra or a body scan.

One relaxes, focusing on the breath for a minute or two. One then shifts awareness to the right hand, each finger. Awareness just rests there for a moment, then the focus shifts to the right arm, then the left: from the right foot leg to the left, then awareness travels up the spine, into the stomach and chest, to the throat and face, all the way up to the top of the head. At this point there is a stillness, and awareness of the entire body. The whole process can take anywhere from five minutes to half an hour; it can be undertaken with or without relaxing background music. I guided Freya and Robyn through a body scan which lasted around ten minutes; by the end of it, I realised they were both asleep.

This is a simple yet powerful healing technique which I hope could be more utilised in hospitals and other healing places. It works as well, if not better, than Panadol.

We are Breath.

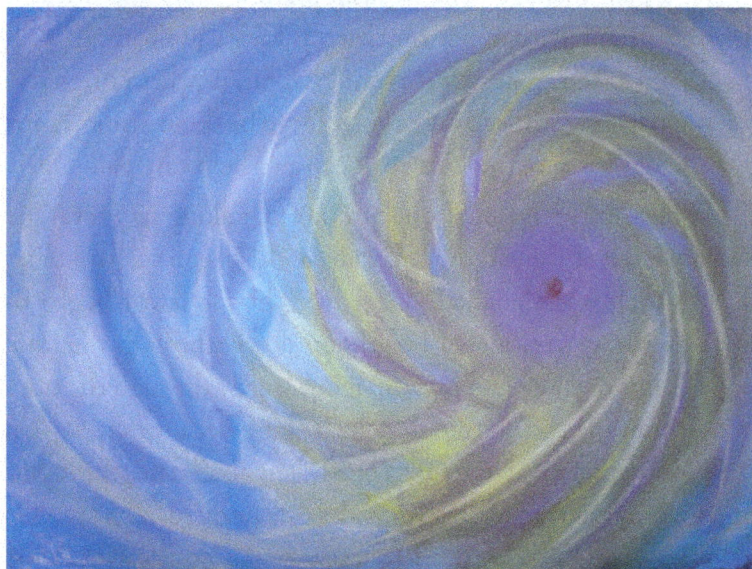

The stillness

EMBRACING THE MOMENT

As I write, I am undergoing physical healing. My bruises and bones are slowly getting better but over the last two years since the bushfires, there have been other bruises of an internal nature, hidden from the world, that could not be seen.

Firstly, there was my year in Canberra, in a cocoon, surrounded by friends, gifts, the creation of a home (temporary though it was); the writing of my first book, *Mallacoota Time*; the beauty of the landscape, the Brindabellas, the Canberra sunsets.

That year, there was also grief, tension, anxiety; relationship issues, stuttering, feeling that everything was surreal. There was a sense of dread about having to make a life choice and ultimately leave Canberra. The dismantling of that nest in Canberra was so hard. I drove around with tears welling in my eyes for a week. Packing our few belongings to move yet again felt like this house too, was burning down in slow motion...

In November 2020 we purchased the house that was to become our new home. Just twenty minutes south of Brisbane City and around forty minutes north of the Gold Coast, we immediately fell in love with the house and location. The house sits in a bush gully, where a creek once flowed. In this little gully we are nestled halfway up the hill, overlooking another.

The sun sparkles each day on the eucalypts and we have many visitors: kookaburras, magpies, lorikeets, currawongs, butcher birds, a few king parrots, wallabies and bush turkeys. The environment is peaceful; we have installed a swimming pool, sun drenched and ready to utilise for at least six months of the year. The pole-frame house is large and airy, made of Cedar, and its large windows and sliding doors allow for soothing cross breezes in the summer.

Arriving in Brisbane was a novelty. There was a sense of adventure and discovery ahead: people to meet, places to see, paths to forge. My family is here now also: my two sons, one in Brisbane and one at the Gold Coast, my two granddaughters, and my father near the city. Our decision to move here felt like the right choice, and in many ways perhaps it is...yet with the last year and a half of Covid lockdowns, restrictions made it difficult to create community networks, travel interstate or even to see family for extended periods.

Gradually music, such a huge part of my life, receded into the background. I got to the point where I felt the wind had been knocked out of my sails. It had been so long since I had performed anywhere, to anyone, that I felt I had lost my ability to do so. I became doubtful and insecure about my abilities. Even when society reopened somewhat, I was too lacking in confidence to seek out performance opportunities. The narrative running through my head constantly was 'I'm too old, I've lost my voice, I'm too out of practice, why would anyone want to listen to me?' On and on it went.

Around the middle of 2022, it began to dawn on me that I was never going back to my old life with Jim: a vibrant tapestry of travel, music performance, community, friendship, nature; of sleeping near a beach, waking to a pastel sunrise and the sound of crashing waves. I began to feel progressively isolated. I was moving into the acceptance phase of grieving. At this point I became aware that the loss that had occurred was a reality: there was no going back. I began to evaluate: had I made the right choice in moving to Queensland? Should we have moved back to Mallacoota? Should I have stayed within my community on the South Coast?

All these questions occupied my mind constantly. I began to wonder who I could call for an impromptu cup of coffee; apart from my own family, and my lovely neighbours, there was no one. This was in stark contrast to my former life in Mallacoota, Canberra and the South Coast, where I could draw on friends at any given moment to socialise with if I felt like it. There had also been a vast network of musicians that I could call upon to perform with, or simply to have a jam. Jim also was suffering from depression and seemed very anxious. He found it challenging to forge any friendships himself, and being of a more reserved nature than myself, did not attempt to go about it. Since his stroke in November 2019, we had not played music together and he seemed to have lost some ability to memorise the music.

So here we were, both feeling trapped on the Island of Queensland, depressed, isolated, and locked down in our beautiful breezy home in this little gully. Whilst we both appreciated the beauty around us, the good fortune of having acquired our new home, and of granddaughters nearby, it simply was not enough to sustain us. We began to suffer once more in our relationship and communication. There were daily misunderstandings and tensions. Our one source of solace was going out on the balcony to feed the birds. It made us feel like we were doing something together that we both enjoyed. It was healing to be able to do what we had done together so many times in our years in Mallacoota...

At this point I contacted the bushfire recovery support worker that had been assigned to us since moving to Brisbane. I explained to her that Jim and I were both feeling isolated and not well psychologically. She said, 'don't feel alone, or as if what you're going through is unusual. We have just had a large call for help from bushfire affected people. It's like a second wave and can happen with trauma around the two-year mark.' She referred us both to a psychologist. During my fortnightly phone calls with the psychologist, I begin to realise that I was living through my memories: most of my waking time involved remembering and grieving for my past life, which I was missing terribly. I began to feel like an old person, sitting on an armchair, reminiscing about their youth.

I had one foot stuck in my old life and one in the new. I understood that if I did not take my foot out of that old life, stepping with both feet into this new life, I would not be able to move forward.

It was around this time that I decided, with the easing of restrictions, to return to Canberra to revisit friends, have the launch of my new album *This Is Now* and take the journey back to Mallacoota for closure.

I realised also that if I did not try to perform music in front of an audience before baring my soul at the album launch in Canberra, I would feel unprepared... So, casting doubts and insecurities aside, and with a feeling of trepidation in my stomach, I called the nearest golf club. I told them that I had heard that they had live music on Sundays, asked if they would consider hiring me for three hours.

I was booked to perform and spent two weeks practising old and new songs that would suit the demographic. Although I was performing other's music, therefore not intimately baring my own soul, it felt incredible to once again reconnect with an audience. People approached me, asking when I would return and complimenting me on my performance or song choices. It reassured me that I could perform at the album launch in Canberra.

The physical bruises are real, but the emotional ones are just as real and hurt just as much. It is only by embracing the moment, that I could begin to allow the emotional bruises to fade.

This is honey for the soul.

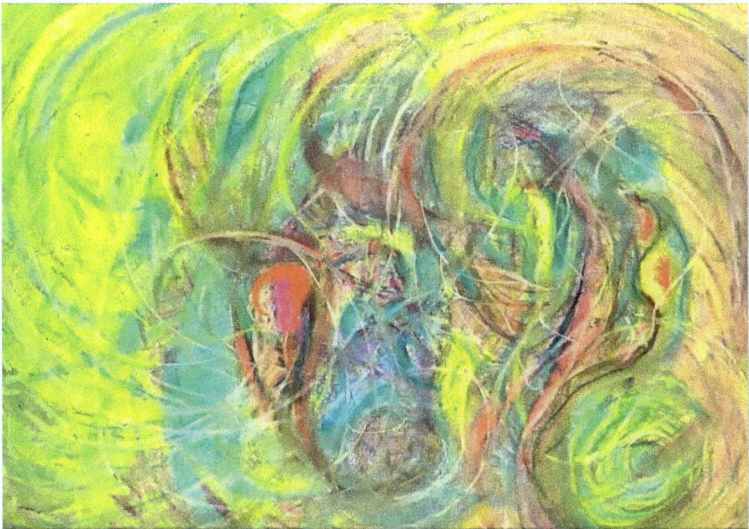

Sun song

SUNLIGHT

I am sitting at home on my balcony, listening to the bird song and allowing the sunlight to soak into my skin. Sunlight is a healer. Vitamin D boosts the immune system, promoting healthy healing of bones. On my recent return to Mallacoota, at the Muddy music night, a woman approached me, handing me a folded piece of paper. 'I wrote you a poem,' she said.

It sat in my bag unread; I opened and read it the following day, in my hospital bed in Canberra. She must have known...

A poem by Rosemary Hannah

The Brilliant Sun
The brilliant Sun
On the horizon
Rising and setting
Earth's star of light.
On the horizon
Colours of light, shining
Earth's star of light.
On the horizon
Colours of light, shining

Earth's star of light
With healing in its rays
Colours of light
Rising and setting
With healing in its rays
The Brilliant Sun.

WATER

Have you ever sat on a balcony or a grassy knoll, overlooking a river, or the ocean, or had a picnic by the lake, and not felt at ease and totally relaxed? Water has this magical quality. it is one of the most soothing elements available to us to be in, on, or nearby. We are made of water; our cells are water.

Since being in Brisbane I have been going to the heated pool for hydrotherapy and swimming. As soon as I am immersed, my aches and pains melt away. Being in the water stills my mind and relaxes my muscles.

In hospital, I could not shower for five days. The day I was wheeled into the bathroom by a nurse to have a shower was a big step forward. As soon as the warm water washed over me, I felt an improvement in pain and mood.

In Brisbane, Jim and I take our granddaughters to the heated pool every Tuesday for three hours. We play, sing, dance, laugh, invent imaginary games. We bond. We are relaxed. There is no tension. There are no arguments, no toys to fight over. There is just water. Beautiful soothing water. To drink eight glasses of water a day is a golden rule we have been taught most of our lives. Pure, filtered water, to cleanse our skin, keep our brains active, nourish our cells, and keep us functioning optimally. Water heals. In it, on it, near it, consuming it. Water is life.

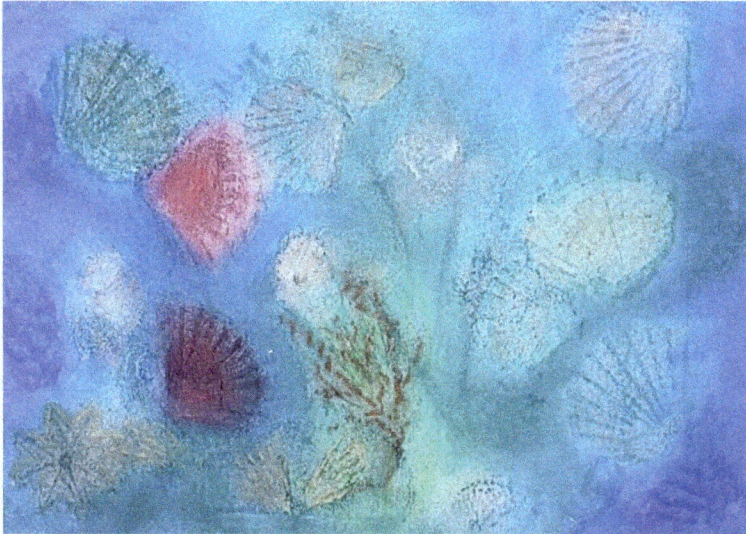

Rockpool

COMMUNITY

Today, for the first time since my accident, I decide to go to the pool. I feel that the warm water will relax my tight muscles, and I know that movement of any sort is therapy.

Since moving to Brisbane, I have found it challenging to find community to connect with. I have missed the community links I had forged on the South Coast, Mallacoota and Canberra.

I arrive at the pool, hobbling slowly on my crutches, feeling trepidation and some anxiety. It is a slow and laborious walk down the ramp. The water is gradually taking my weight, I am now waist high.

There are ladies in the water doing hydrotherapy. They wave at me, smile.

They ask me what is wrong, why I am on crutches, where I have been...

I tell them I have suffered an accident, broken my hip, been in hospital. These ladies, they gather around me, smile; I tell them my story, they listen. They are compassionate, offer advice, words of encouragement, a helping arm.

'Take care Milena, just take it slow'...

'You'll be ok Milena, you're a strong woman'...

'Don't do too much, just let the warm water heal you'...

They walk at my pace; they keep an eye on me. *They care*... When my body is tired and I decide to end the water session, they congratulate me:

'You did it!'

'Well done! '

'you'll be back to swimming in no time!'

I hobble painfully up the ramp and suddenly I feel two of the women by my sides:

'You look like you're struggling' they say. 'Hold onto me'.

So, I take their arms, put all my weight on them, and take a step. I feel the weight lift, the worries dissipate, the pain ease.

These sisters, helping me up the ramp out of the pool, are likely not aware of the magnitude of what they offer: for the first time, since arriving in Brisbane, I feel the sprouting seed of community...

ART

In the hospital next to me Freya is drawing. She is an artist; her speciality is portraits. This is what makes her tick. It is who she is, as music is a part of who I am. In the bed opposite me, Robyn is colouring. She buys children's colouring books, and spends hours colouring them in, relieving and distracting her of her inability to breathe properly.

I am engulfed suddenly one day by a desire to draw in my hospital bed. I ask Robyn if I can borrow her colouring pencils. In my bag I find a black ink pen. I start to draw, become so absorbed in my task I forget who I am, or where I am. I simply am. I call the picture the sharpness and softness of experience.

I am home now, in my bedroom, healing. I spend long hours in bed, the most comfortable place for my body now. My view is the bamboo outside my bedroom window and in front of me, on the wall, a work painted for Jim and I by a Canberra friend after we lost everything. It tells a whole story -a man and a woman standing outside their gypsy caravan on green grass. It is a starlit night; their horse is camped nearby. The man is strumming a guitar, and the woman is standing by his side entranced, listening.

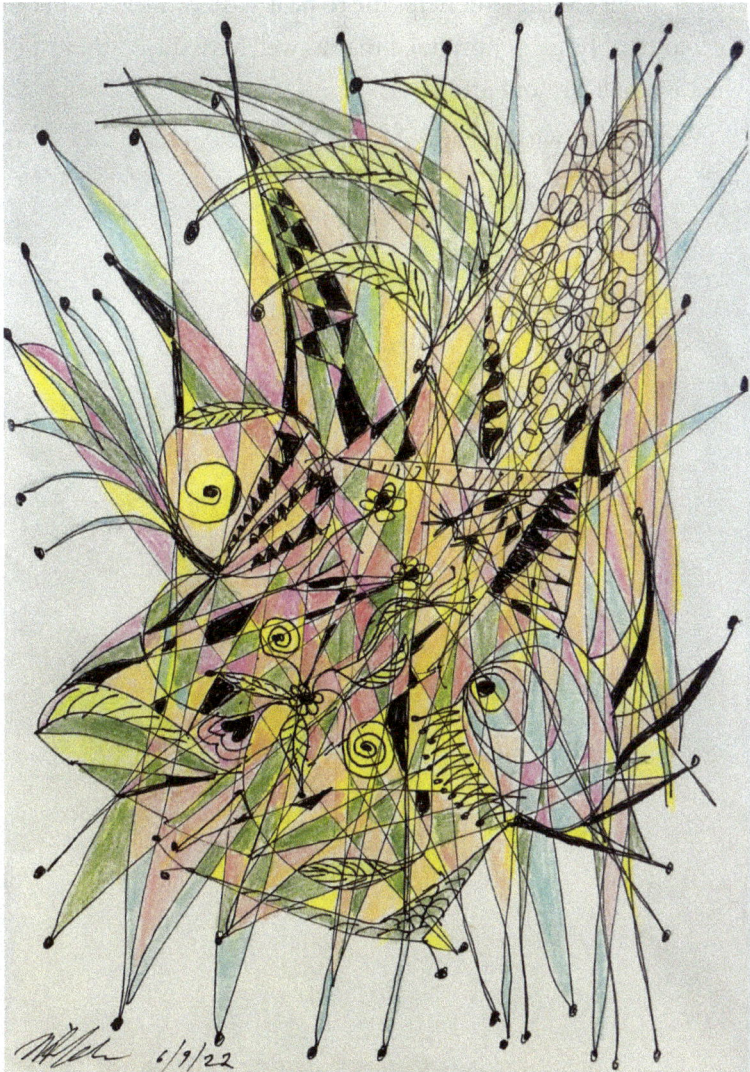

The softness and sharpness of experience

I spend a long time looking at this painting, this gift from my friend, and it soothes me, helps me to heal. If this wall was blank, as they invariably are in hospital, I may as well have stayed there. For what is a wall without art?

What is life without art?

CHILDHOOD

I remember how it felt to be a child: do you? ... there was no ego, no worry, no thought of future; no sleepless nights pondering tomorrow's tasks; simply existing: watching the ants crawling on the concrete, absorbed in their activity ... I spent hours playing, splashing in puddles, laughing at the joy of it all. I lay on my stomach drawing pictures from my imagination, of owls palm trees princesses fairies and desert islands....

I tripped and hurt myself: my mother would hug me, clean the sore and kiss it better... I went to the hospital for stitches or to have my tonsils out: it was no big deal, I had no fear about it: I knew I would be alright, and I was. Post operative jelly and ice cream healed all. So, with a free mind the body could use energy for healing, and did so swiftly, because there was no anxiety linked to the situation.

Thus, I returned to my world, in the moment, drawing snails in bowler hats, playing in the waves on a sunny day, saturated in joy. It is not until today, years gone by, that I invest my energy in worrying about what the future holds ... strangely, the more I fret the less I enjoy life.

In my healing process, I am now trying to reconnect with the child in my heart: I still my mind, focus on my breath, the breeze, the present; let everything else take care of itself. I surrender.

I could read every book under the sun, study every text on healing: or I could watch my granddaughters, two and four, and learn to be in this moment, the sun shining down on the me that I am.

I am learning.

SWEET CHARIOT

The day after my birthday in February 2022, Jim departed for Sydney to pick up his yacht *Sweet Chariot*, in Botany Bay, and to sail it home to Brisbane. He left with the words 'I'll be back soon. I'll see you in eight days.' He flew to Sydney with a crew member who was to sail back with him and went aboard his yacht.

Around the 23rd of February 2022 a weather system arrived across the eastern seaboard of Australia almost as devastating as the bushfires of The Black Summer 2020. These were to become one of the nation's worst recorded flood disasters. They spread from south-eastern Queensland right down to the mid Coast of New South Wales and onto Sydney.

Brisbane experienced widespread flooding. Over the course of the floods twenty people lost their lives and the property damage in Queensland alone was estimated at $2.5 billion. The relentless flooding caused food shortages due to farmers losing crops, as well as the ground being so saturated that even a small amount of rain put many areas at risk of further flooding.

The first night the rain started I could not believe that so much water could fall from the sky. It was heavy and constant. It never let up. I would wake and think 'it must stop now' but it would just continue.

The morning came and still it rained, all day and the next night also. It rained like a biblical deluge. Our pool started to overflow. Water began flowing down our driveway and puddles and ponds began to appear in the garden. Roads closed all around. Brisbane River rose and burst its banks. I was alone.

Jim was on his yacht in Botany Bay waiting to return home. I began to have visions of the house tumbling down the hill in a muddy landslide. There had in fact been other landslides in the area and I suppose because I had been involved in one natural disaster, the thought of being in another was not impossible to conceive.

Jim was unable to return home because the crew member that had accompanied him to Sydney decided to opt out. Sailors were communicating with each other, advising that it may be dangerous to sail with the volume of debris that was washing out into the ocean from Moreton Bay.

Jim decided to wait and search for a new crew member to accompany him on the return trip to Brisbane. Eventually he found one who suggested that they should sail eighty kilometres out at sea to avoid any debris and Eastern Ocean currents. Days became weeks. Finally, after seven slow motion weeks, Jim and his crew member decided on a favourable weather window and set sail for Brisbane.

Jim kept in touch quite regularly via telephone, but there were often many hours where I did not hear from him. Almost eight weeks to the day that Jim had left Brisbane, he called me, asking if I could pick him up from the Port of Manly at 1am the following day. I agreed to do so. The following day arrived. I called Jim at around 10 pm to make sure he was on course, and ready to arrive. There was no reception, and I could not get through. I tried again at 11:30pm and again at midnight. There was still no connection. I tried once more at 1:30 am but was unsuccessful. I decided to get a bit of sleep and wait for them to contact me. At that point I was quite concerned, but not overly worried.

I woke at 8 am and immediately called Jim. There was no response. I tried again at 9am and at 10am. At this point worry started to set in. I was extremely concerned that something untoward had happened to them. I called the water police and gave details of the yacht's name and crew members names. Water police informed me that they would start a search; they were quite concerned. I spent four or five long anxious hours awaiting their call. Finally, the phone rang, interrupting the heavy silence.

Water police informed me that they had been successful in locating the yacht. Jim and his crew member had encountered difficulties at Amity Point, having to reroute, going around Stradbroke Island, further North to Moreton Island, and docking at Manly, extending their trip by a further ten to twelve hours. I later learnt from Jim that the crew member had decided against Jim's instructions to cross the South Passage bar at the Northern tip of Stradbroke Island at Amity point, at around 2am the previous morning. Jim had been sleeping in the cabin below and the crew member was on watch. The bar is notorious for being dangerous and unpredictable; attempting to cross in a new yacht, without previous experience posed extreme risk.

Jim awoke with water coming in below, and objects on the yacht flying in all directions. He was slammed against the wall. He managed to climb up onto the deck and saw that the crew member was crossing the bar. The yacht by this time had broached and was at risk of being smashed against the ground. Jim ordered the crew member to exit the bar. The yacht recovered an upright position again. The crew member made a second attempt at the bar against Jim's instructions: again, they were pounded by enormous waves and once more the yacht broached. Jim described the whole ordeal as terrifying explaining to me that he very nearly came close to drowning twice.

The experience left Jim with a sense of anxiety; for myself it was an ordeal, left alone to experience the stress of the floods, coupled with the fact that my partner was sailing eighty kilometres out in the ocean with a stranger. I do believe that both Jim's near-death experience, as well as my own brush with death, being trapped under my own rental car, has left us both with symptoms of post-traumatic stress disorder. It is only through communicating with each other about these ordeals, and the limitations they have left us with, that we may begin to relate better, and to heal.

Since our challenges began, our relationship has suffered: yet it survives! I contemplated how it would feel to lose that love, imagining our love lost...

Quiet Night of Stars
A quiet night of stars
A moon of gold delight
An orchestra of waves
A symphony of Love
A look you gave to me
That stopped my beating heart

And then you held me near
On this quiet night of Stars...
your lips so warm on mine
A feeling so divine
I thought our love would last
But now it's in the past
I walk the sand alone
My lips have grown cold
Our footprints washed away
On this quiet Night of stars...

THE PASSAGE OF TIME

All things shall pass...

The deep raw wounds on my feet where the gravel tore at my skin is starting to dry up. The black bruising around my ribs has almost faded. The swelling and pain in my hip is lessening. The bone is beginning to mend. The trauma of the bushfires is fading like my bruises. Time does not negate pain. It does not erase trauma nor dull grief. It only serves to dilute their essence: their rawness, immediacy, urgency. Where I sit today, with my crutches by my bedside, is not an indication of where I will be sitting in three days, months, years, decades.

I try and remind myself of this. Time heals all wounds...

GRATITUDE

Jim tells me that we used to work on projects together, in our pre-fire life, but feels this is now lacking. This makes him sad. I agree that life has somewhat narrowed upon moving to Brisbane. I reflect on how we can begin to recreate that feeling of working together towards a goal; whilst we may not be able to plan a long trip far away, or perform at a big music festival now, there is no reason we cannot break our future goals into smaller parts: we can plan an overnight trip to the Sunshine Coast hinterland; we can practice three songs to perform at a casual musical evening; we can take a ferry to one of the surrounding islands for a picnic.

I tell Jim that we must practice gratitude. We can focus on what we have, not what we do not have; we can strive to see beauty in any situation rather than despair. We can reflect, each day, on what we are grateful for: for this home together, for each other, for our family nearby, for the birds that visit our veranda each morning...

My bones hurt and my bruises ache. Every part of me hurts. I struggle on my crutches and feel despondent at the inability to take a few steps unaided. My emotions are fragile; I cry easily, tire quickly. Then, I remember this:

I am fortunate to have survived. I am grateful.

A PERSPECTIVE OF LIFE FROM A WHEELCHAIR

It is Spring. Today, I want to hire a wheelchair. I wish to go out, immerse myself in the violet beauty of the Jacaranda blooms that paint Brisbane purple in springtime.

Although I want this, I feel trepidation: I somehow feel that relying on a wheelchair is a sign of weakness on my part , a sort of ' giving in'; but I cannot contemplate hobbling painfully through vast parks on my crutches.

I pay my deposit and we transfer the wheelchair into the car. We stroll along the river, under the jacaranda trees, life in slow motion. I breathe in birds, flowers, clouds; hordes of people at a Sunday morning market. I smile at people and meet their eyes. Some are uncomfortable and look away. Others return my smile ...

After this first, unfamiliar experience of being pushed in a wheelchair, I begin to utilise it more regularly: for shopping, attending live music, going to the park; I begin to see it as a pathway to recovery and freedom. It allows me to get out and live life fully. It provides me the opportunity to engage socially and to interact with others.

Being in a wheelchair may not necessarily mean that the occupier is ' wheelchair bound', or permanently disabled. Many people choose to use a wheelchair only occasionally, when they may be experiencing worse pain than usual; most importantly, many people, myself included, may be using wheelchairs as part of their healing journey. I know that for me, to be able to be outside under the purple jacarandas is a simple yet powerful step toward my recovery . Being in nature, smiling and having others smile back, is participating in life. This is an immeasurably valuable part of my healing journey.

The wheelchair is my sweet chariot.

ACCEPTANCE

Anyone, at any time, can be thrown a situation that is distressing and traumatic. Jim's stroke, the loss of our home, my recent accident, are all situations which occurred instantly, changing our lives.

Jim knows this truth well, having been thrown from his motorbike in 1986, and suffering two years in hospital and very nearly losing his leg. Trauma can be alleviated by accepting change, however hard that may be. ... Change is inevitable; time cannot be rewritten. I can go over the moments before my accident, torment myself with would haves and should haves, but it cannot alter my reality. Far more beneficial to accept what has happened, learn from it, and move on.

Conserve energy for healing by practicing acceptance. I remind myself: To swim against the current is harder than flowing with it...

PURPOSE

Even with the limitations of my mobility, and my occasional feelings of despondency, I continue to try and have purpose. I compose music; I look after my granddaughters; I water the plants; I spend time with my elderly father; I make a meal for my partner. It hurts to stand and chop carrots, but I do so with love. It hurts to drive the forty-five minutes to pick up my granddaughters; but I do so with love. It hurts to get in and out of the car for my father; but I do so with love. It hurts to bend over and water the plants; but I do so with love.

Perhaps it would be far easier to sit on the couch and let my feelings of despondency take over: but in the laughter of my granddaughters, the moments of connection with my father, the tending of a plant, the care of my partner, I am living. Living and healing. And in doing so I am caring for me.

HAPPY ANNIVERSARY

Today marks one year since my car accident. The trauma rears its sinister head, dark and foreboding, slowly wrapping its tentacles around my body and soul. My mind goes over events of that life changing day methodically, in technicolour precision:

10.30am leaving Mallacoota

5.00pm approaching Canberra

5.13pm stopping to photograph a staggeringly beautiful sunset.

5.14pm parking in driveway, exiting car, removing luggage.

5.15pm car rolling backwards, dragging me down the driveway, trapping me under it.

5.20pm sky darkening, three degrees, drizzling. still

trapped, still in pain ...

Etcetera ...

Today, at 5.13pm, a year to the day of my accident, I mark the moment by finding a vantage point to take a photo of todays beautiful sunset. This simple ritual reminds me that the sun will rise and set, rise and set, and do so again; it reminds me that there is always beauty. It marks that I have survived, and commemorates how far I have come, how much I have achieved...

I can get caught up in the memory of staring death in the face; it was very traumatic. Alternatively I can celebrate: last night I had an amazing album launch, and got on and off stage on my crutches; I can walk a few steps unaided, I can cook meals. I can drive. *I'm alive*! So much to be so thankful for!

Celebrating the small wins is a path towards healing ...

Happy anniversary to me.

HOME

I think, just perhaps, I have finally come to understand what home means. It has taken me a lifetime to be able to define it in words.

Home—a place you return to where everything feels 'just so'. A comfortable, soothing place, a refuge, where everything is how you would like it to be; every picture hung where you want, every cup stored just the way you like; every piece of furniture arranged in a way that suits you; every pillow fluffed up perfectly. However comfortable another's home is, or even a hotel, it is never the same, because that sense of *just so* is lacking.

In our forest gully home, I sit on my pink, white and blue peacock-print armchair, gazing out at our sun-drenched wooden deck across to trembling bamboo leaves against a blue Brisbane sky. I know I walk the healing road, and though the path may sometimes be convoluted, the destination is always in sight. This precisely because of the sense of being home. Surrounded by nature and birds, my cat Pushki, by music, art, and sunlight; keeping an inner sense of faith, practicing an outward expression of gratitude. Breathing in love. Everything is just so. I am going to be alright.

THE NOW

I am taking a shower. Getting in and out is hard. I have a shower stool to sit on.

The hot water rushes over my skin. I look down and think ' I HATE WHAT I HAVE BECOME'.

But it's not me I hate. It's my disability.

It's knowing that I can't just get out of the shower easily and get dressed and go for a walk in the sunshine.

It's knowing that every step is painful.

It's knowing that I can't reverse what has happened.

It's knowing that these crutches that I have been dragging myself around on for ten months now, have become a part of my life and that I must depend on them.

It's knowing that there is a possibility that this is as good as it gets.

I swing between anger and sadness.

I practice whispers of acceptance and gratitude but then a voice louder than those drowns them out.

There is a sense of foreboding about my future.

I try and practice being in the moment.

Right now all is well. I cannot change my past and I can't control my future.

I finish my shower, slowly dress myself and go outside to sit on the sunny verandah. I slow my breath. I hear butcher birds singing their song, and the breeze gently promises me that this moment is perfect.

This moment.

This Is Now

That was then and this is now,
Time fast forwards,
don't know how,
But the music in my heart
goes round and round
And the leaves in the breeze
make the same sound
That was then and this is now,
let it go and take a bow,
For the stage is set to do it all again,
This is now and that was then
It will all come back to me,
Life is one big mystery,
That was then and this is now
That was then and this is now,
From today I make a vow
to breathe out old, and breathe in new,

fresh and cool as morning dew
It will all come back to me,
Life is one big mystery,
That was then and this is now...

EPILOGUE

It is May 2023: it has been nine months since my accident.

Just as a baby in the womb grows over the term of the pregnancy, so do my bones, muscles, nerves, emotions.

It has been a long slow road, and it is not over: in fact, it has only just begun, as I tentatively begin taking my first few steps unaided.

Finally, finally, after eight months of dragging my tired body up and down, back and forth on crutches, every cell in my back, arms and feet hurting, I can stand on my feet, put one in front of the other. A small miracle.

My body is getting stronger.

I have been swimming each day , at first dragging my legs behind me, then tentatively kicking, and now , able to swim thirty laps of freestyle.

My body says thank you.

———

My mind is not at peace though ...

Today I feel frightened.

Driving on the freeway, I have a sudden panic attack. Heart beating, palms tingling, breath quickened.

I lose connection with my legs, as though they are invisible.

I feel light headed ...

Returning home, I am tired. I toss, turn, restless, unable to sleep. Finally, I doze, awaking fitfully, body buzzing with anxiety.

I finally drift off, dream about driving with Jim back to the South Coast. We reach a mountain top. The vista is awe inspiring, the vast blue ocean spread out before us ...

Suddenly, I see congestion on the road below us: cars are backed up. I put my foot on the brake but cannot reach it. The car is rolling out of control down the hill. We are going to crash and die!

I awake in terror, sweating, heart racing...

There are other moments that terrify me; a simple manoeuvre such as parking my car.

A car is reversing out beside me. I feel that I am rolling forwards out of control. There is a pole in front of me: I think I will smash into it. I begin to cry, terrified. But the car is not rolling. It is stationary. I am perceiving movement as the other car backs out, yet it is only an illusion.

Jim reassures me, ' it's ok we are not moving.'

At that point, not only am I in the grip of blind terror, but also the realisation of how easily triggered I have become. I realise I am a fragile soul at risking shattering.

This provokes further fear.

I begin to cry despairingly, big gasping sobs. It takes me ten minutes to settle, calm my breath ...

I lose a part of myself as

I go into meltdown ; but actually I find a part of myself :

In that moment I am a terrified little child trying to protect myself. I reconnect, wrap my arms around her, whisper 'it will all be okay'...

———

My psychologist says I display post traumatic stress disorder:

I am so easily triggered; my sleep is disturbed by dreams of being out of control or of rolling forwards .

I carry my scars outwardly, yet I am also hiding them inwardly.

Anxiety , depression, and PTSD are all normal responses after trauma.

I will walk side by side with Gratitude in the coming days and months grateful that I have a psychologist, provided with strategies to deal with anxiety such as breathing, meditation and visualisation; grateful for my ability to play music; it is unwaveringly my grounded space; grateful for my cat. I stroke her and her purr calms me. She is my happy place; grateful for the continuing gift of life; for the opportunity to evolve and offer support to others by having gone through my experiences.

In the end, I am grateful for my trauma.

It makes me stronger.

It makes me who I am.

One foot forward ...

ACKNOWLEDGEMENTS

In the creation of *One Foot Forward*, I have first and foremost to thank my friend Peter Gamble for his expert design and guidance with the manuscript.

I also wish to thank Kim Hollingshed for the beautiful foreword she has gifted me. Also to my friend Ranjan Chadhauri, who has always supported me as a writer, and to my friend Anne Finlay, who has offered her lovely words for the back cover.

I thank Marcus from Echo Books for publishing my second book with them.

I thank my family:

My sons Bryn and Louie for their unwavering love, my parents for the same, and my partner Jim Horvath for caring for me so tenderly over the course of a year as we have travelled this healing journey.

I thank life itself for what it has offered me, both joyful and traumatic. In the richness and depth of my experiences, I evolve as a person with more compassion, kindness, and understanding.

The heart, broken into pieces, comes together stronger, more resilient and more whole.

Thank you, the reader, for accompanying me as my journey continues, one foot forward.

Milena Cifali

www.ingramcontent.com/pod-product-compliance
Lightning Source LLC
Chambersburg PA
CBHW071101090426
42737CB00013B/2426